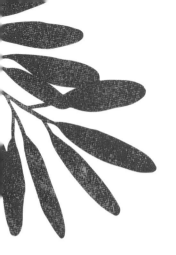
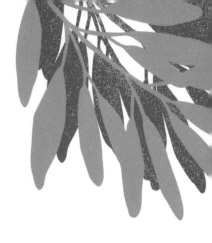

Transitions
4th
Trimester
Journal

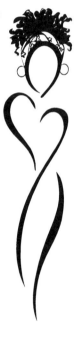

Transforming

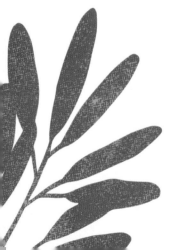
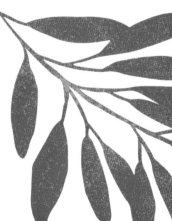

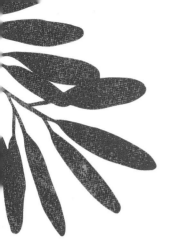
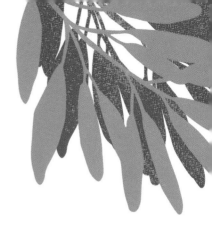

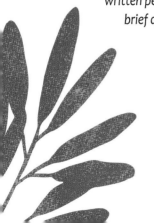
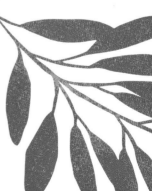

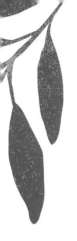
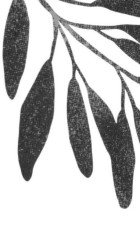

This journal belongs to

_____

Motherhood is a story you will
write for your child. It's the
beginning of their biography.

Once upon a time...

_____ was born

Date   _____

Time   _____

Weight   _____

Length   _____

_____

_____

_____

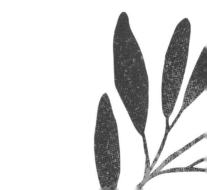

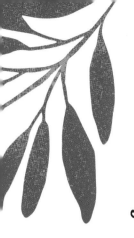
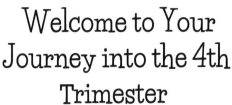

Welcome to Your Journey into the 4th Trimester

This journal will take you into

uncharted territory, no two pregnancies

are alike. It's your story to reveal

Welcome to yours

First Congratulations Mama

You are a rock star !!!
Carrying a life and
giving birth teaches you
about a strength that you
didn't even know you
had.

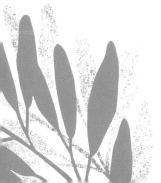

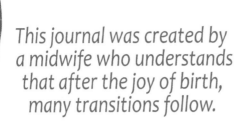

This journal was created by
a midwife who understands
that after the joy of birth,
many transitions follow.

There are many changes
that can occur due to hormones,
sleep deprivation, and
emotions that can range from
joy to stark terror.

This journal was designed to
support this transitional
time, and give you a place to
write your joys, fears,
triumphs, and gain
confidence.

This will be a self-care
guide, as well as a place to
find affirmations, and just
plain reassurance.

Motherhood doesn't come
with a manual, but during
the next few weeks, you and
your baby will get to know each
other well. Your schedule
will begin to regulate.

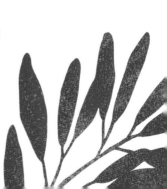

5

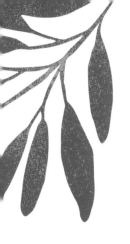
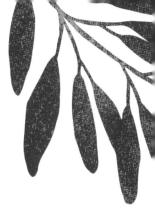

Important Numbers

Midwife/MD _____

_____

_____

Doula _____

_____

Nurse _____

_____

Lactation _____
Consultant

_____

_____

_____

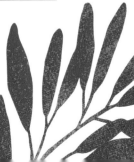

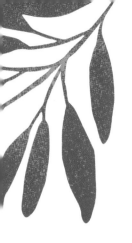
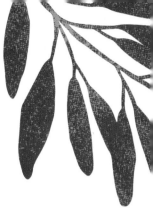

When to call and follow up

Call if:
Temperature 100.4
Pain upon urinating
Abdominal pain
Headaches

If you are sad, and crying, not
eating, or able to sleep

Call 911 if you experience:
Heavy vaginal bleeding
Swelling of face or hands
Any chest pain
Shortness of breath
Dizziness
Fainting

Call if you are not feeling like
yourself, or if you feel something
is just not right.

You know your body better than
anyone else. If something doesn't
feel right, call your provider

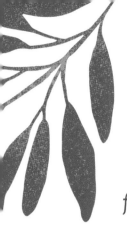

Notes
for your visit to your provider

I delivered my baby on _____. (date)

My last period began on _____. (date)

I have been feeling _____

_____

_____

_____

I am concerned about _____

_____

_____

_____

_____

I know my body and _____._____doesn't feel normal

What could this _____mean?

The medication(s) I am taking are:

_____

_____

_____

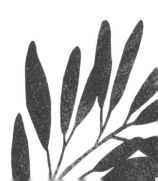

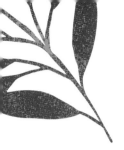

Things to Do when you are feeling stressed

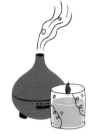

Turn on your aroma diffuser/candle

Put on some music and dance

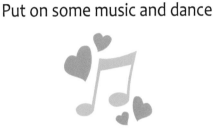

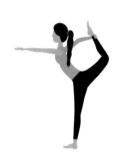

Alittle stretching

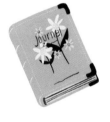

Write down your feelings in this journal

Have a cup of tea

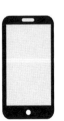

Call a friend

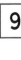

I Care for Myself Spiritually ...

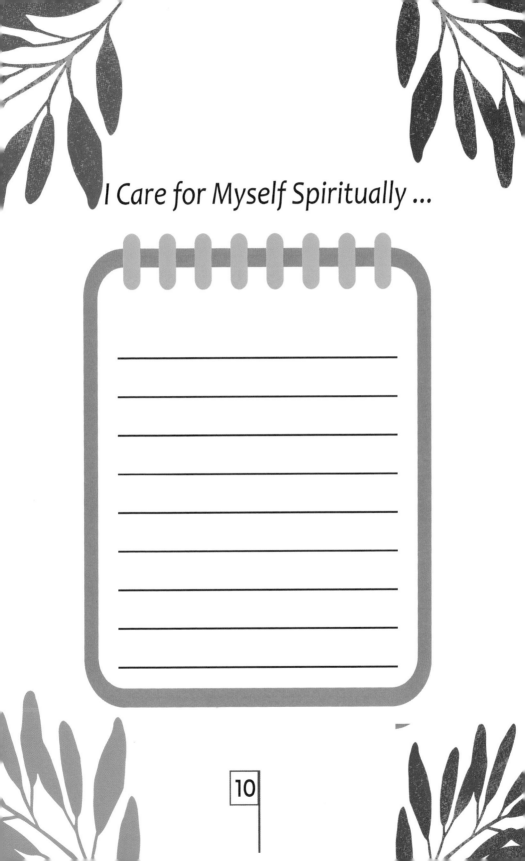

I Care for Myself Physically ...

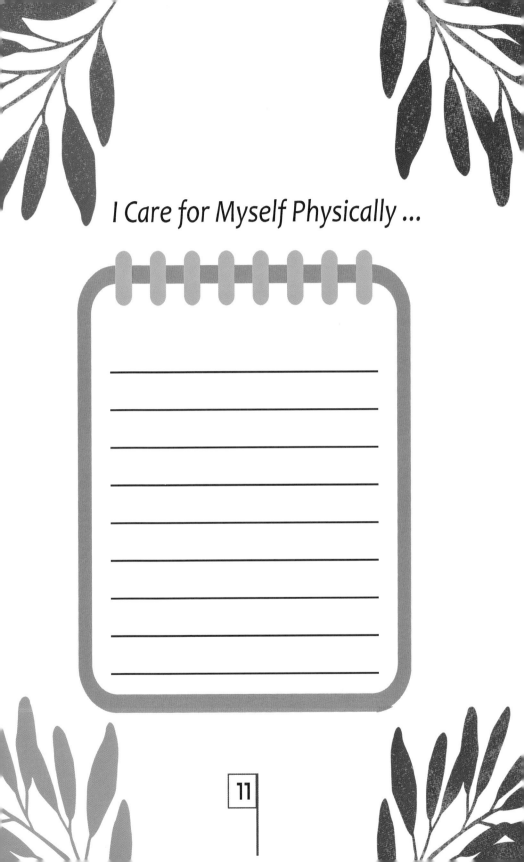

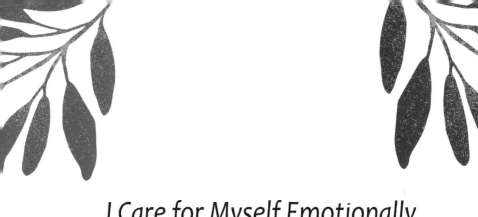

I Care for Myself Emotionally ...

_____

_____

_____

_____

_____

_____

_____

_____

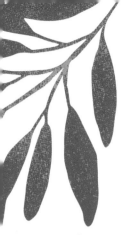
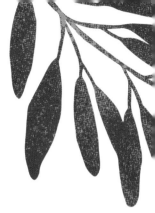

Affirmations

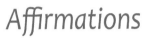

I am powerful, and I am capable of great things.

I am equipped, I am enough.

I am a responsible adult. I can do this, I will add
my own flavor and flair to it.

I will make some mistakes everyone does; my baby
will grow up knowing I love them, and did my best.

I will learn to laugh at myself, and enjoy this
exciting journey called parenting.

There are many options, I can be brilliant,
creative, loving, and unique. There is no one else
on this earth just like me.

My baby will be blessed, my household will be
blessed, my partner will be blessed
Amen.

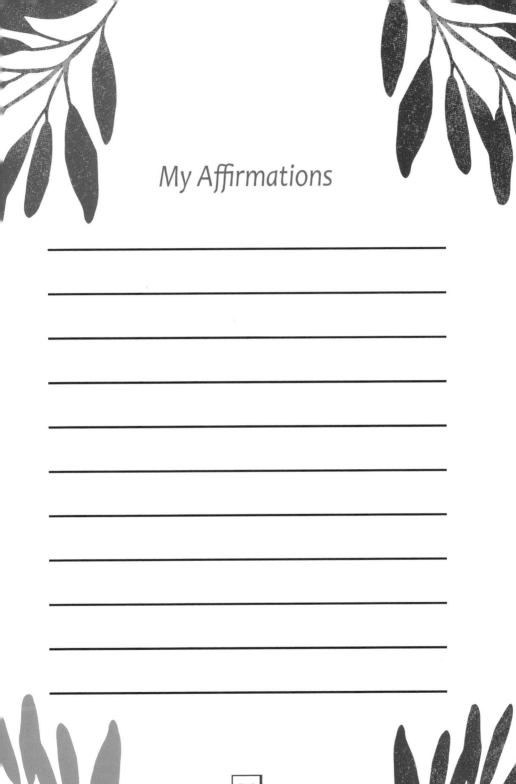

My Affirmations

_____

_____

_____

_____

_____

_____

_____

_____

_____

_____

My Affirmations

_____

_____

_____

_____

_____

_____

_____

_____

_____

_____

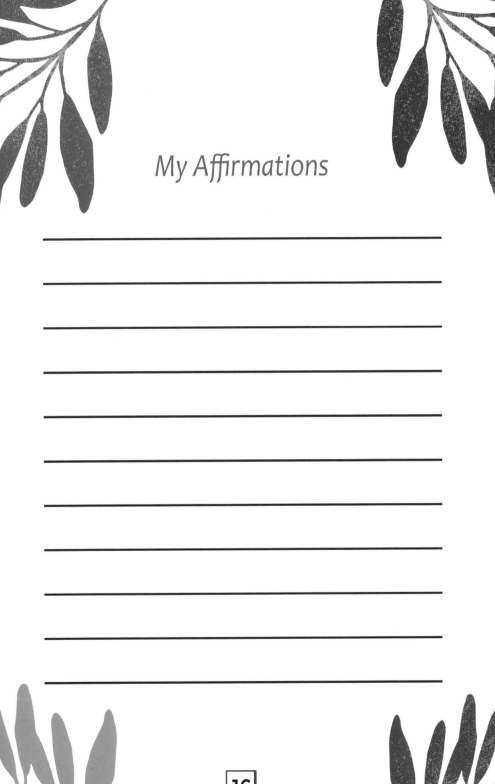

My Affirmations

_____

_____

_____

_____

_____

_____

_____

_____

_____

_____

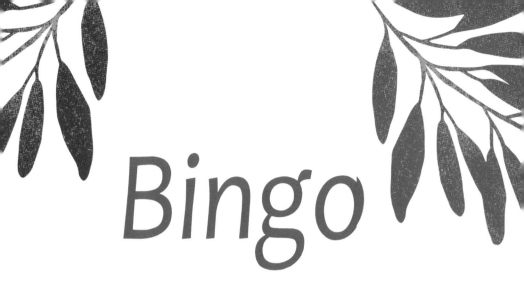

Bingo

SHOWER	GOT DRESSED	CALLED A FRIEND	PROCESSED MY FEELINGS	COMPLIMENTED MYSELF
EXERCISED	MEDITATED	CAUGHT UP WITH FRIENDS	SPENT TIME WITH MY PARTNER	LISTENED TO MUSIC
TOOK A BREAK	DRANK WATER	Free	TOOK A SOCIAL MEDIA BREAK	TREATED MYSELF TO A FACIAL
TOOK A NAP	GOT 8 HOURS OF SLEEP	TAMED NEGATIVE THOUGHTS	WATCHED A MOVIE	HUGGED BY BABY
TOOK A FEW DEEP CLEANSING BREATHS	SPENT TIME WITH NATURE	DECLUTTERED MY SPACE	WROTE IN MY JOURNAL	COOKED A HEALTHY MEAL

17

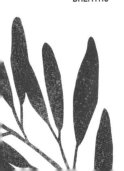

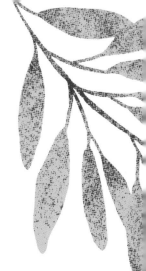

THE FIRST 12 WEEKS

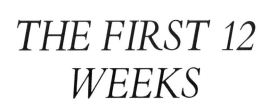

- [ ] Read one book

- [ ] Meditating or Deep Breathing

- [ ] Begin a gratitude journal

- [ ] Be patient with myself

- [ ] Recite 2 affirmations daily

- [ ] Take a 15 minute walk 3x a wk

- [ ] Get comfortable breastfeeding

- [ ] Do something relaxing each day

18

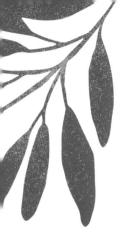
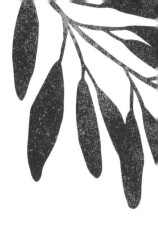

If you find you're
feeling anxious, and
depressed ask for help
from your partner,
family, friends, or your
provider.

You're not alone...

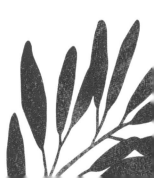

Things to celebrate today...

_____

_____

_____

_____

_____

_____

_____

_____

_____

_____

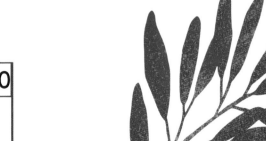

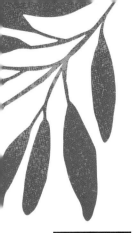
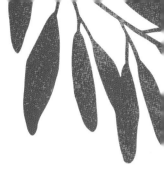

word find

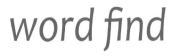

The 4th Trimester

```
B  B  T  W  K  M  K  B  F  K  D  W  W  T  M  L  Y  J
M  I  V  R  V  L  N  Q  M  I  D  W  I  F  E  A  L  E
Y  O  R  B  A  Q  P  F  D  S  G  G  O  U  Q  C  A  P
B  B  T  T  A  N  E  H  C  H  A  N  G  E  A  T  F  Y
R  A  M  H  H  F  S  S  E  L  F  C  A  R  E  A  M  I
E  B  F  V  E  Y  A  I  F  A  N  R  J  D  V  T  A  L
A  Y  Q  A  E  R  K  T  T  C  L  H  R  O  Z  I  M  R
S  Q  D  I  M  P  H  B  I  I  E  T  G  U  O  O  A  T
T  G  K  X  Y  I  F  O  F  G  O  B  H  L  U  N  J  L
I  A  S  O  X  Y  L  J  O  F  U  N  F  A  R  U  I  U
E  N  Q  X  X  F  V  Y  X  D  V  E  Y  T  B  Q  P  G
M  N  U  D  A  N  X  S  L  E  E  P  H  Y  J  W  A  F
```

Find the following words in the puzzle.
Words are hidden → ↓ and ↘ .

BABY	FATIGUE	SELFCARE
BIRTH	HEALTH	SLEEP
BREAST	LACTATION	TRANSITION
CHANGE	MAMA	
DOULA	MIDWIFE	

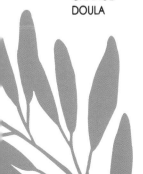

I'm grateful for ...

Write a word each day to describe how you are feeling.

word of the day

I had an AHA
moment when . .

_____

_____

_____

_____

_____

_____

_____

_____

_____

Don't believe the hype...

Looks can be deceiving
Motherhood is not easy...
but it's so rewarding
It's okay to ask for help

_____

_____

_____

_____

_____

_____

_____

_____

_____

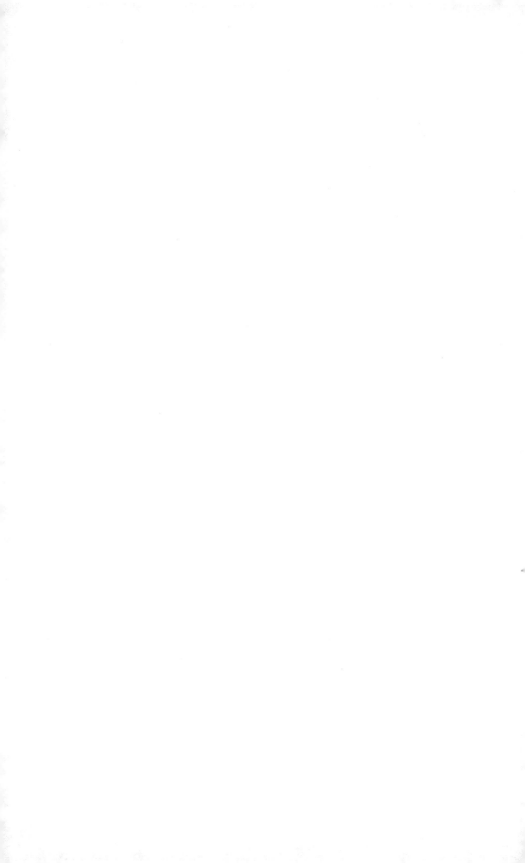

My superpower is ...

_____

_____

_____

_____

_____

_____

_____

_____

_____

_____

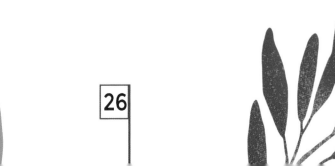

YOU'RE AN
AWESOME MAMA

_____

_____

_____

_____

_____

_____

_____

_____

_____

_____

You've got this... it's all good
It's okay to do it your own unique way

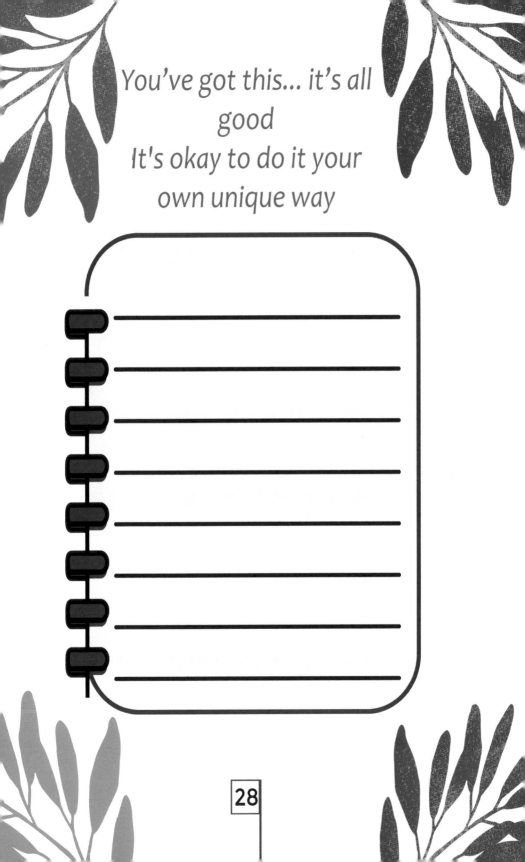

Today I will ...

_____

_____

_____

_____

_____

_____

_____

_____

_____

_____

_____

_____

_____

_____

_____

_____

_____

_____

_____

_____

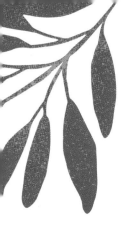
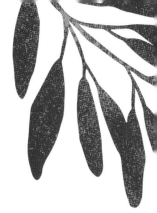

Word find answers

```
B . T . . . . . . . . . . L . .
M I . R . . . . M I D W I F E A . .
. O R . A . . . . . . . . . C . .
B B T T . N . H C H A N G E . T . .
R A . H H F S S E L F C A R E A M .
E B F . E . A I . A . . . D . T A .
A Y . A . R . T T . L . . O . I M .
S . . . M . H . I I . T . U . O A .
T . . . . I . O . G O . H L . N . .
. . . . . . L . O . U N . A . . . .
. . . . . . . Y . D . E . . . . . .
. . . . . . . . S L E E P . . . . .
```

Word directions and start points are formatted: (Direction, X, Y)

BABY (S,2,4)	FATIGUE (SE,6,5)	SELFCARE (E,8,5)
BIRTH (SE,1,1)	HEALTH (SE,8,4)	SLEEP (E,8,12)
BREAST (S,1,4)	LACTATION (S,16,1)	TRANSITION (SE,3,1)
CHANGE (E,9,4)	MAMA (S,17,5)	
DOULA (S,14,6)	MIDWIFE (E,9,2)	
FAMILY (SE,3,6)	MOTHERHOOD (SE,1,2)	

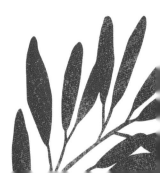

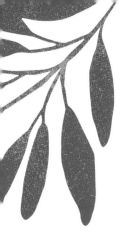
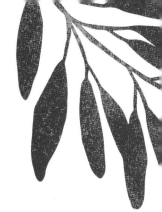
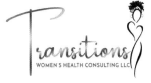

Food for thought in a world full of options...
Dr. J

www.transitionswomenshealth.net

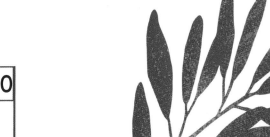